Advance Praise for Postcards from Oncology

"***Postcards from Oncology*** made me laugh about cancer. It lifted me up to a place of not-so-quiet joy and demonstrated a suspiciously healthy approach to dealing with serious illness. Bill's letters are a primer for how to be a successful patient (read: 'co-healer') and should be required reading for anybody in the medical profession—not to mention anyone with a life-threatening illness. Bill Raines is that rare phenomenon we all long for more of: *A Good Example.*"

Greg Tamblyn
Speaker, Singer, Songwriter, Humorist
"Saving the World from Whiney Victim Love Songs"
http://www.gtsongs.com

"Reading ***Postcards from Oncology*** was so delightful! From a nurse's point of view, it was not only humorous for the staff … but certainly a positive way for Mr. Raines to keep his spirits up and to assist in his recovery."

Jane Ryan, R.N.

"Bill's book is wonderful. It is guaranteed to make you laugh and lift your spirits, regardless of what is frightening and challenging in your life. Let your healing and liberation begin with laughter."

Barbara Sherrod

POSTCARDS FROM ONCOLOGY

One man's light-hearted version of being a cancer patient

BILL RAINES

ISBN # 0-911041-22-2

OPA Publishing, a division of
Optimum Performance Associates
Box 12354
Chandler, AZ 85248-0023
Email: info@opapublishing.com
Online at: http://www.opapublishing.com

Printed in USA

opa

Dedication And Acknowledgments

This book is dedicated to my wife, Sat Atma Kaur. I married you as Sandy and I now recognize you by your spiritual name, which means "Princess with the true soul." You are a most delightful life-partner in the dance of life. May you accept your own magnificence, which is so apparent to me and many others. I am a man who is so very blessed, and you are the most precious of them all.

I wish to thank my brother in Spirit, Joel Baehr, Minister at Unity of Mesa, who has shown me the path of joy and gives me a place to make a difference in the lives of others.

I also thank all of you who read my email medical musings and encouraged me to write this book. You are all so beloved to me. I wouldn't have done it without you.

Finally, I wish to thank my editor/publisher, Paul McNeese, who put ***Postcards*** in book form for me and brought it to the world. You made it easy, Paul.

Bill Raines
June, 2004

Preface

"I am here to shine the light of my heart on those longing to be more light-hearted."

This book has not been written just for cancer patients. It is for anyone who longs to be more light-hearted and take life and themselves less seriously.

My perspective is that what happens in our life is not nearly as important as how we respond to what happens. Christopher Reeve comes to mind as one inspirational example.

My own personal example was Ken Keyes, Jr., author of *Handbook to Higher Consciousness*. My ex-wife's comment the first time she met him was, "That man is so radiant that you need sunglasses when you are around him." He also happened to be paralyzed from the shoulders down all of his adult life, the consequence of polio when he was in his twenties. I spent a week learning from him in 1983, and I never saw Ken without a twinkle in his eye. His energy was joyful and light-hearted throughout the week.

I was a different person after being with him. I could no longer justify either feeling sorry for myself or taking too seriously what life put on my plate. On May 14th, 2003, what life handed me was THE BIG C. That was the day on which I received the results of a biopsy that revealed cancer on both sides of my prostate. We would see how radiantly joyful and light-hearted I would remain now that the "fit had hit the shan!"

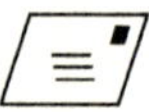

We humans are, if nothing else, predictable. When something that matters in life goes wrong, the mind will surely wrap itself around that circumstance. A life-threatening health challenge, loss of job, discovering that our child is taking drugs or our spouse wants a divorce—anything that threatens the status quo will provoke fear, foster anxiety and destroy our peace of mind. As quickly as the negative thought arises, we will very likely become joyless and will begin to invest a lot of time and enormous amounts of mental energy writing, producing, directing, editing, and projecting sad or scary mind-movies about the future.

At my first radiation treatment visit I had a profound awakening. I was on the radiation table, lying on my back with my pants and undershorts down around my knees. A woman I had never seen before had put a block between my feet and tied them together; she was going to take some x-rays. All at once a most unexpected thing happened: I had an almost irresistible urge to giggle or burst out laughing. The scene seemed so bizarre and humorous to me. I didn't giggle, but I *did* start having an imaginary conversation in my head with the radiation therapist. I imagined myself to be a writer for a situation comedy on TV.

Postcards from Oncology

At that very moment, I decided I'd deal with the whole process of my cancer treatment program by observing it in a humorous way. I'd be the comedy scriptwriter, playing it for laughs. Almost immediately I began to feel a lessening of tension, and I realized that I loved imagining strange and often unprofessional conversations with the staff, some of whom did not exist. Once I got on a roll, I even started imagining conversations between the equipment and me.

I have an email list of several hundred people who have taken "Power of Now" classes with me or have been participants in my "Living Love" group (check my website at http://www.billraines.net). When the word got out that I had cancer, many of these folks wanted to know how I was doing, told me they were praying for me, or wished me well.

What a great audience! I decided to start sending out what I called my "*Postcards from Oncology*."

The response was tremendous. Many people told me that they started looking forward to a periodic "postcard" from me. A number of them encouraged me to get these medical musings to a wider audience in book form (and this is it).

I also gave the radiation therapists copies of each email, which became a part of my medical file and eventually led to an interesting conversation with my radiation oncologist, as you will read about later.

It is important for me to mention two things right away and before we get into the "meat" of the book.

First, let me emphasize that the members of the medical staff were, in fact, impeccably professional and competent. They were also very caring and delightfully pleasant company. I think of them with respect and gratitude. I even miss them. And second, I have not used the real names of any of the medical staff in my postcards, since it is not always easy to discern what is real and what is imagined, and I certainly wouldn't want to inadvertently embarrass anyone.

Furthermore, if one is in physical pain, or if the quality of one's life is severely diminished or gone, it is not a laughing matter. In no way do I intend to disrespect or minimize that truth for anyone who is in that situation. I hope that my musings will bring some smiles and laughter and reduce self-created emotional suffering for any reader who is facing a difficult challenge in life. I also wish the same for their loved ones. I surely would have been less light-hearted through this process without the complete love and support of my beloved wife, Sat Atma. It is to her that I dedicate this book.

Following the ***Postcards*** section of the book I will offer some personal thoughts on how we all can celebrate more and struggle less in this wonderful adventure called "life."

Remember: Be silly.

Bill Raines

Postcards from Oncology

August 1, 2003

Greetings, Friends.

Some of you know that I had my first radiation appointment today. To keep all of you posted on my experience I offer the following:

All oncology patients are given an ID card with a magnetic strip that you slide through a machine when you arrive in the waiting room. Soon thereafter, someone will come out to escort you to the treatment room or you'll be paged over a speaker system and asked to come back to treatment.

In my case, perhaps because it's my first visit, a nice lady comes into the waiting room, smiles at me and says, "Mr. Raines, we have been expecting you. Come with me."

As we enter the treatment room, my attention goes to a table that looks hard, with a very large machine hovering over it.

"Mr. Raines, I need you to drop your pants and under shorts and lie on your back on the table."

"Gee whiz, we just met. I don't even know your name yet."

"I'll protect your modesty, Mr. Raines," says the nice lady as she drops the towel on me just where I most want her to drop it.

"I don't have any modesty."

"Good. We should get along fine. I'm going to put a block between your feet and tie them together."

"Do you realize how long it has been since I have been tied up by a woman while in a prone position?"

"My guess would be quite a long time, Mr. Raines. Now I'm going to take this marker and place some marks on your body. They won't wash off."

"Please don't write your initials on me; I'm a happily married man."

After marking me in several rather "delicate" places, she puts the marker away and picks up a measuring device.

"I need to take some measurements, Mr. Raines."

"Yeah, I remember one night in Hell Week at my fraternity when I was a pledge and they did some measuring. The guy with the most impressive measurement got to wear a Fire Chief's hat and was thereafter known as "The Big Chief." The guy with the least impressive measurement was forever known as "The Jockey."

"Were you The Jockey, Mr. Raines?"

"CERTAINLY NOT!"

"It's the depth of your body and pelvis we are measuring. It helps us draw a bead on your prostate when we radiate you."

"Good idea. The adjoining territory is quite dear to me. Let's keep it out of the line of fire, shall we?"

"We do our best, Mr. Raines."

Meanwhile, the big machine comes down on my left side, moves up above me, then down on my right side. To keep from feeling like a deer in the headlights I start singing softly, "Om Namo Bhagavate Vasudevaya."

"Nice tune, Mr. Raines. What do the words mean?"

"They mean that I am one with the heart of the Lord in the radiation machine."

"Mr. Raines, I don't think that the heart of the Lord is *in* the radiation machine."

"Oh, but you are wrong. God is everywhere, in everyone and everything. Eckhart Tolle writes that even a stone has some consciousness of God in it."

"Tolle?"

"Yes, he wrote the book, *The Power of Now*. I teach a class called "Living the Power of Now." It's based on his book. I am singing to the machine that I am one with him and I love him."

"Good for you, Mr. Raines." Short, pregnant pause, then…"Did you know that we have psychological consultants on call and available to our cancer patients? Sometimes the stress and worry over having cancer affects their thinking. I'll speak to the doctor about it."

Well, anyway, by this time we're done, so I don't have to respond.

"It was certainly *interesting* to meet you, Mr. Raines."

"Wow, this is a piece of cake. My chanting worked really well. I didn't feel a thing."

"That's because we didn't do anything, Mr. Raines, except take measurements, shoot some pictures, and complete the setup. We'll begin radiation next Wednesday."

"You mean all this was for nothing?"

"We won't send you away empty-handed. Here is a parking permit that allows you to park in any of the spots reserved for Oncology. Just put it on the dash of your car."

"Thank you so much."

As I walk through the parking lot to my car, I notice all the cars that have an Oncology parking permit on the dashboard. I realize that I am now part of a very special group of people. Maybe you're part of that group, too—in one way or another.

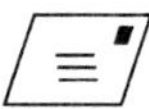

Postcards from Oncology

August 12

One of the procedures of the Oncology Department is that when you are called back to the radiation room you must tell the radiation therapists your date of birth on each and every visit. So when I get there I call out, "3-28-27," and only then am I admitted into the inner sanctum.

While I'm lying on the table, my mind starts to wonder why this procedure is necessary, especially since I've already been there several times. Do they need security measures to keep people from sneaking in to get their body zapped with radiation? I don't think so.

Now, I ask myself, who would this experience appeal to? That's a tough one. Let's face it, when the treatment's going on you can't see, hear or feel anything. Hmmm.

Got it!! It's the flashers they want to keep out! The payoff is that you get to drop your pants in front of two women at one time and not get arrested for it. In fact, they actually *ask you* to do it. Five days a week, no less. A flasher fix—every day. Wow, cool, man!

Postcards from Oncology

Can't you just imagine it? I drive into the Oncology parking area and immediately spot a couple of guys just hanging around. As I'm getting out of my car the first man approaches me and says, "I'm looking to buy some information, dude."

"What kind of information?"

"Like your name and date of birth."

Before I can answer, the second guy shoves the first guy out of the way.

"Whatever he offers to pay you, I'll top it."

Before any money changes hands a third guy runs up.

"Hey, you guys, don't bother. I got in this morning with a black market date of birth, and when I dropped my drawers, they just dropped a towel on me. Didn't even take a peek. Even worse, they were totally indifferent."

Then I hear another voice—not in my mind. It's Lucy, my radiation therapist. Oh, well, back to reality.

"We've finished for today, Mr. Raines. How was your treatment?"

"Wonderful, as always, Lucy. See you tomorrow."

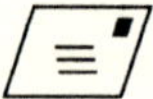

Postcards from Oncology

August 14

At the hospital, the most direct route from the parking lot to Oncology is through the Maternity Center. I'm starting to experience side effects from that. I had morning sickness this morning, and my contractions are now 30 minutes apart. If they come any faster I may have to find another route to Oncology.

Another problem. A little jealousy has developed between my radiation therapists. The other day in one of my postcards I mentioned Lucy—but not Lois. Lois is feeling left out. Let it be part of the public record that I was intimate with Lois before I was with Lucy. Lucy was on vacation when I started treatment. To avoid further complications, I also want to mention Pat, who comes in on Thursdays and Fridays to tie my feet and drop the towel.

Each Wednesday I get to meet with my oncologist. Our conversation usually goes something like this:

"Hi, sport, how are you doing?"

"So far so good."

"Nothing to this, Bill, right?"

"Well, I can see that talking to me once a week doesn't put much of a strain on you."

"Wise guy, huh? I like that. Now give us a view of the target area."

(Pants dropping time again—this time in front of a man.)

"Whaddya mean 'us,' doc? You're the only one who can see back there."

"That's right, sport, and nothing has fallen off yet."

"I didn't know that was one of our goals."

"Always read the fine print on the Permission to Treat form, Bill."

"Wise guy, huh? I like that."

"Bill, you've had five treatments, so you probably will start having some bowel symptoms."

"Shhhhhhhhh!"

"Shhhhhhhhh?"

"My bowel can hear that."

"Your bowel can hear what I'm saying?"

"Yes it can, and I don't want you giving it any bad ideas."

"Let me get this straight. You believe that your bowel can hear?"

"Certainly, and I don't want it to get any negative messages."

"I see. This is sort of like your heart connection with the radiation machine. The therapists told me about that."

"*Exactly*. Now you understand."

"I see. By the way, Bill, did you call for an appointment with our psychologist?"

"Hey, doc, I *am* a psychologist."

"Really . . . and you help people with their mental problems, right?"

I smile. "Right."

"Well, we can all take comfort in that, Bill. Unless there is something more I guess we are done for today."

"Thanks, doc. I'll see you next Wednesday."

"Actually, Bill, I have some vacation time I haven't used. I think I'll take a vacation day next Wednesday."

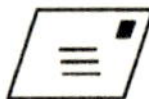

Postcards from Oncology

August 20

All right, all right, so it's been a while since I wrote. I've been experiencing writer's block—although I'm loose (very loose!) in some other ways. More about that later.

However, my radiation therapists are threatening to boycott my treatment if I don't have another postcard in my hand when I arrive tomorrow. By the way, if you're finding my writing too explicit for your taste, let me know and I will eliminate (love that word!) you from the mailing list.

As I arrived yesterday:

"Hi, Mr. Raines, do you have plenty of gas?"

"That's very personal, Lucy . . . but no, just some fatigue."

"I meant for your car, silly, what with the gasoline shortage and all. By the way, our other oncologist wants to see you after your treatment today, since your doctor is on vacation."

So, after the treatment, into the doctor's office I go.

Postcards from Oncology

"How are you, Mr. Raines? I see that you've completed eight treatments."

"I'm doing quite well."

"Mr. Raines, I want you to turn around, drop your pants, bend over and moon me."

Right away I can tell that this doctor likes me more than my regular oncologist. I comply.

I hear the witnessing nurse whisper, "Cute butt."

"Thank you. Sat Atma has always told me it is one of my best features."

Now the doctor has another request. These guys are never satisfied.

"I want you to spread your cheeks, Mr. Raines."

I would really prefer not to be liked this much by him.

"Everything looks fine, Mr. Raines."

I wonder if the cavity searches are to prevent me from smuggling drugs into Oncology? Or maybe it's part of a program to generate empathy for prison inmates (I feel your pain, guys)."

Postcards from Oncology

On the way home my bowel starts letting me know that he is not a happy camper.

"Hey, man, I don't like all of these radioactive bullets you're sending in my direction."

"What can I say? Talk to my prostate. He's the cause of all this."

"Are you serious? That loser is toast. We are all distancing ourselves from him as much as possible. By the way, Bill, how is your sex life?"

"Nobody likes a smart ass; we're not going there."

"Well, I'm just letting you know that I can't take care of business in a normal fashion and dodge the radiation at the same time."

"I understand. What are my choices here?"

"Constipation or diarrhea—take your pick."

"That's a no-brainer. I pick diarrhea. Think of all the money I'll save on colonics."

"Whatever you say, boss."

As I'm driving home from the hospital in Sat Atma's car (mine is low on gas, Lucy), I turn on Greg

Tamblyn's CD. The song "Heart of the Mother" comes on and I sing along:

I am one with the heart of the Mother.
I am one with the heart of love.
I am one with the heart of the Father.
I am one with God.

Tears of gratitude start running down my cheeks as I sing. I feel so very blessed each day of my life. I have so many wonderful friends who love me and to whom I can write just like this. Thank you all for being a part of my life.

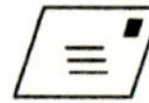

Postcards from Oncology

August 25

"Come on back, Mr. Raines, I'm ready for you."

"Lois, where's Lucy?"

"She's not here right now. She may return before we finish."

"I am accustomed to a ménage à trois, Lois. This won't do."

"You're spoiled, Mr. Raines." Offering me a small rubber circle, she says, "Would you like to hold this while I radiate you?"

"Nothing less than a stuffed animal will do."

Lucy enters.

"Lucy, I expect you to be here as well as Lois for the daily unveiling."

"I know, Mr. Raines, it won't happen again. Well, we're finished. Remember, it's your day to see the doctor."

Postcards from Oncology

In the doctor's office:

"Well, Mr. Raines, how is your stream?"

"A little cold for skinny dipping, but the trout are biting."

"I was referring to your urination, Mr. Raines."

"Free and easy. Flomax is a great drug."

"Good. Now turn around, bend over, and moon me."

I comply. I always comply.

"Fantastic, Mr. Raines, simply fantastic."

The two nurses are nodding in agreement.

I turn around, blushing. "Gosh, really?"

I leave with the most energy that I have had in some time.

Sidebar note: My acupuncturist sold me some herbs that the Chinese use to reduce the side effects of radiation. I know they're powerful herbs because I can't pronounce my "r" sounds anymore.

Postcards from Oncology

This week my most embarrassing moment comes when I attend the Board of Directors meeting at my church, Unity of Mesa. The problem is that I'm spending too many of my waking hours lying face up on a table. I lie down at Oncology every day, at my acupuncturist's office twice a week, and when Carla and Caroline do their energy work. Our board meeting takes place in the minister's office around a large table. I walk into the meeting, and before I know it I'm climbing up onto the table to lie down on my back. In the process, I knock off a dish of mixed nuts. The board members immediately take a vote and decide that I *am* one.

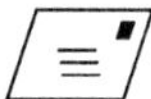

Postcards from Oncology

September 2

Friday, August 29th, I arrive at the hospital, drive into my usual parking place and there, on the Oncology Parking sign, sits a large black crow. In my mind I immediately hear the opening music from the HBO program "Six Feet Under." It always opens with a picture of a crow sitting on the edge of a grave. I hate that music. "God, could you cut me a little slack here?"

As you know, all of us cancer patients report to a room where we wait to be called over the speaker to come back to the radiation room. The most frequently heard phrase in my life these days is, "Come on back, Mr. Raines."

And, as you can imagine, there's not a lot of eye contact, conversation, or laughing going on in the waiting room among the patients. Only the staff is cheerful and upbeat.

I walk in, sit down, and say out loud, "Well, here we all are, another day in paradise."

I remember farting in church one time as a teenager. The reaction here turns out to be quite similar, except for one lady. She looks over at me, makes eye contact, and smiles.

Shortly thereafter, I hear that old refrain, "Come on back, Mr. Raines." I stand up and say to the other patients, "My time to shine." As I walk out, the lady who smiled at me says, "Shine on, Mr. Raines."

All right!

In the inner sanctum:

"Good morning, Mr. Raines, how are you?"

"I don't like having a black crow perched on my parking space, Lois."

Chuckling, she responds, "You mean like on 'Six Feet Under?'"

"Darn right! It sets a bad tone for this otherwise joyful experience."

Both therapists start to giggle as they tie my feet and maneuver my body into the line of fire.

"Hey, it's easy for you to laugh. I'm the deer in the headlights here."

More laughter.

"Okay, that's it. I'm not coming in for treatment on Monday."

I don't know if they rehearse for these moments, or what, but together, as one, they answer, "Well, Mr. Raines, if *you're* not coming, then neither are we."

Radiation vacation for Labor Day.

Meanwhile, back at the ranch, my diarrhea has moved into full bloom—at least that's my fervent prayer. If, by any chance, this is only *half* bloom, then my clients will have to start coming to my house for their sessions. In fact, I'm soaking in the bathtub as I write this. Plans are being made to move one of the TV sets and a VCR into the bathroom.

I mean, I don't mind this so much when I am at home. However, I hate that when I'm playing in a poker tournament at the casino I'm the only person who needs to bring a box of "Flushable Moist Wipes" to the poker table. For me, the phrase "Don't leave home without it" no longer brings MasterCard to mind.

When a good day in your life centers around your bowel and your bladder, you can be sure that the quality of your life has gone downhill.

Postcards from Oncology

I remember taking an undergraduate college course in Abnormal Psychology. The professor was discussing our psychological stages of development according to Freud. Freud stated that some people who were fixated at the "anal stage" of development could find a good bowel movement more satisfying than having sex. My thought at the time was, "Either those people don't know much about making love or I don't know how to have a great bowel movement." Alas, I am coming to a new awakening of what Freud was talking about.

Tomorrow is going to be another big day for me. After radiation, I'm scheduled to go to my urologist for my second implant of a hormone pellet. The hormone decreases the production of testosterone and slows the cancer's growth. I will have three of these implants over nine months. They are making me impotent—but the good news is, I am more in touch with my feelings, ladies.

There's no problem on the home front—unless my breasts get larger than Sat Atma's. She won't stand for that. In the meantime, we share our hot flashes together.

Postcards from Oncology

We celebrated our 13th wedding anniversary yesterday. We agreed that we would rather have a wonderful, loving, affectionate, harmonious relationship without sex than to have great sex in a loveless, combative marriage. To any of you who have a harmonious relationship and great sex, I can only say, "I hate you."

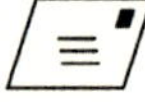

September 3

Wednesday. Visit the doctor day! As I enter, he's holding my medical file.

"Mr. Raines, you have quite a sense of humor. And I do find some of your emails amusing."

"But?"

"But . . . some people reading them may form the wrong impression of our staff and the treatment program."

"It's all tongue-in-cheek, doc. You know that."

"I do know that, and you know that, but some readers may not. They might think that we're not being professional in our comments and our behavior. That's all I'm going to say about it."

"I understand your concern, and I *will* get a disclaimer out."

Reflections afterwards:

The fact is, at least two readers actually *did* believe that the staff had suggested that I see a psychologist.

You'll meet a psychiatrist in a little while, but he exists only in my imagination.

The entire medical staff has been impeccably professional in their every word and deed. We *do not* have the goofy conversations that I hear in my mind and write to you.

Why am I writing, anyway? First, it's great fun, and it's tremendously therapeutic for me. Second, I want to put them together one day in a book for others who may be facing a tough challenge. However, I, in no way want to give people a false impression about the very wonderful people who help those of us with cancer.

I as finish writing this postcard, I realize how much more fun it is to write the silly ones.

After I sent this postcard out, I received many emails in response. Here are a few samples:

Dear Brother,

How terribly important your silly memos are. I could not have been more depressed and down today. Then, your postcard arrived and I had a wonderful full belly laugh. I don't think that your book would be just for cancer patients, but rather, for anyone who needs a good laugh.

Keep your magic coming, laugh angel.

S. K.

Dear Bill,

WOW!! I am really disappointed that your adventures in Oncology are not real. I figured that you were just the person to bring some perspective, joy and light into that setting. Please tell me that THIS email is the make-believe one.

Barbara

Hi Bill,

I love the way that you are using humor to move through the challenge. In sharing this, you are showing us that there are many ways to deal with the hand that we are dealt in life. I love getting the postcards, keep on stretching that imagination.

Bev

So I continue to write the emails and share copies with my radiation therapists. They continue to place copies in my medical file. There's never been another word said to me about them. My oncologist and I have a great relationship. Even when he expressed his concern with me, he did not do it in a scolding way, nor did he ask me to cease and desist. Perhaps, the disclaimer was sufficient to address his concern.

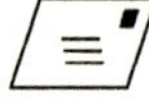

September 4

How do I love me? Let me count the ways:

Daily, I swallow the following:

HydroEye	4 tablets
Flax Oil	4 tablets
Flomax	1 tablet
Methel-tetrahydrofolale	1 tablet
Indo-3-Carbinol	1 tablet
Ginger	1 dropper
Astagelus Ligustrum	6 tablets
Calcium Citrate	1 tablet
Omega Plex	3 tablets
Core Plex	3 tablets
Ditropan	1 tablet
Prilosec	1 tablet

Fortune Delight w/SunnyDew	2 quarts
VitaShake w/Quinary	2 packets
Vitadophilus	1 packet

Best of all, I get hormone injections. You don't even have to swallow this one. They inject it into your abdomen every three months. Try it fellows, and you, too, can have hot flashes with your wife. And you'll be able to think with your big head all of the time.

I had a big day planned today, and by the time I finish swallowing all of this stuff to give me more energy, I am so tired that I'm going back to bed. I lie down, and here come the voices again, starting a conversation in my mind:

"Stop complaining! Bill Romanoski takes over 100 supplements a day."

"Yeah, but he wants to play in the NFL and break someone's eye socket. I just want to teach a class."

"What the hell ever happened to good old steak and potatoes?"

"Not a healthy diet."

Postcards from Oncology

"How about a cheeseburger and fries? I haven't had a cheeseburger in ages."

"We don't do red meat anymore."

"It's not red, it's brown."

"It's red before they cook it, idiot."

"Okay, a banana split then. I haven't had a banana split in a coon's age."

"Dairy products are a no-no, and cancer cells love sugar."

"You've got to be kidding me. Cancer feeds on sugar?"

"So I've been told. Stop whining and drink your VitaShake."

"Okay, okay, then how about some sex? It's not red meat, and there's no dairy or sugar involved. I can hardly remember what an orgasm is like."

"I know, buddy. We need to have a talk. Remember when you used to play golf. You loved that, right?"

"Yeah, man, those were great times. I played two or three times every week."

"How long has it been since you played golf?"

"About 30 years."

"Do you miss it?"

"Nope, but I remember it fondly when I drive past a golf course."

"Right, and you sold the clubs because you knew you weren't going to use them anymore, right?"

"Right."

"Well, I've got some bad news and some good news. The bad news is, you are likely to play 36 holes of golf in one day before you have sex again. The good news is, you can remember all the fun you and Sat Atma have had every time she walks by *and you don't have to sell your equipment.*"

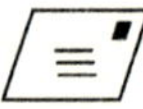

Postcards from Oncology

September 9

Greg Tamblyn was in town this week performing at our church. He is partly to blame for this writing I'm doing.

In the very first email that I got from him, he signed off telling me, "Be silly." His most recent one was signed, "Cause trouble." So, I have gotten more and more silly and it is causing more and more trouble.

Anyway, he told me that he is hooked on getting these postcards and hasn't received one for several days and he is beginning to experience withdrawal symptoms. This one is for you, my friend.

They told me last Friday that they wanted to do a cat scan on me today. For a moment, I considered showing up carrying Bandit, our Siamese cat, for the scan. However, reason quickly prevailed. (Greg, there is a limit to this silliness stuff.)

So, after my radiation treatment, two women, one on each side, have me by the arms and escort me upstairs for the CAT scan. I feel like a fugitive being taken into the courtroom. When I get on the table three of them work to get my body lined up just so.

"Don't try to help, Mr. Raines."

I'm to let three women have their way with my body? That brings new meaning to the word "surrender" for me.

I'm fascinated that as the machine is taking pictures of my innards a "smiley face" light comes on. When it's finished taking its photographs, a "sad face" light comes on. Amazing! I guess this machine really loves its work.

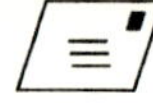

Postcards from Oncology

September 10

When the alarm went off at 6:45 this morning, I realized for the first time that I really didn't want to go in for my treatment. I was up most of the night communing with my bowel. I got very little sleep.

Well, at 7:05 the phone rang. It was Lois from Oncology:

"I have some bad news for you, Mr. Raines."

Believe me, the last words you want to hear from Oncology are, "We have some bad news for you."

"Gulp."

"We have to cancel your treatment today. The machine is down, so we will see you tomorrow."

Wow! If that's bad news, I wonder what they would consider good news? I smile and go back to bed, secure in the knowledge of how powerful my thoughts have become. I don't want to go in for treatment today, so the machine hears me and breaks down. Are that machine and I of one mind, or what?

Later that same morning I told our minister this story. All he said was, "I'm not messing with you, Raines."

To check all this out, I decided to have a conversation with the machine:

"Hey dude, why aren't you working today?"

"I can't hack all the rejection, man, so I said, 'Screw it, I'm not working today.'"

"What rejection?"

"Yours, man. You couldn't stand to come down here with me for even 15 minutes today. I'm sick of all this negative energy directed at me."

"Whoa, buddy, you're taking this way too personally. I had a sleepless night last night. It's nothing against you. In fact, when I watch you do your work, I'm impressed."

"Don't b.s. me. You're counting the days until you're finished with me. I'll prove it. How many treatments so far?"

"Twenty-one."

"And how many left?"

"Seventeen, maybe eighteen."

"I rest my case. You are counting because you want to be done with me. Everybody does. I thought you were different, telling those folks that we were one in the heart of God. No one ever said that about me before. Then, this morning you reject me, too. That's the last straw."

"Listen, I'm a therapist, and people don't want to come back and see me either. They get rid of me a lot quicker than anyone gets rid of you."

"They do?"

"Absolutely. No one ever comes to see me five days a week. Not one person, ever. Yet, I don't take it personally. It's the nature of our business. Our clients are in pain, and they want us to get them healthy and pain-free. Then, they don't need us anymore and they move on. That's a good thing."

"What about that guy in your class that didn't like that you decided to come to me for help?"

"Well, some people think that your methods are harmful, and they think that they know better ways to fight cancer. Don't worry about it! You know, for a machine you're much too sensitive and co-dependent."

"So, you don't have anyone to hang around with you?"

"Well, actually, I think my wife is with me for the long haul."

"There you go, man. I've got no one but my patients." *. . . Long pause . . .*

"Have you checked out the cat scan machine upstairs?"

"Say what?"

"She's magnificent, and she has a smiley face you wouldn't believe. She's quiet, capable, and she brings in the big bucks, too. To me, she looks like everything a radiation machine could wish for in a significant other."

"You really do care, don't you, Mr. Raines?"

"Just call me Bill. Remember, the Lord works in mysterious ways. I'll see you tomorrow. I need your help in finishing off this cancer."

"I'll be here. See you tomorrow, Bill."

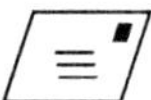

September 12

"Good evening, my fellow Americans, this is Walter Cronkite, bringing you another 'Eye on America' report. Once again, we are traveling across the country to find a human-interest story to bring to you.

"Since there are millions of you with cancer, tonight we bring you the story of one man's battle with prostate cancer. This is the story of Bill Raines of Gilbert, Arizona. I interviewed Bill and some of the other people around him to bring you this story."

"Jill Ross, I understand that you were with Bill on May 14th when he received the results of his biopsy?"

"Yes, Bill was counseling me when the call came in on the speaker phone in his office. The urologist told Bill that he had bilateral prostate cancer and that he needed to come in to discuss treatment alternatives. Bill agreed to call the next day to make an appointment."

"What did Bill say to you after he hung up the phone?"

"He said, 'Now where were we, Jill?' It was like he had just heard the weather report instead of receiving a cancer diagnosis. I couldn't continue with our session, but he seemed fine."

"No reaction at all to getting the bad news?"

"None. It blew me away."

"Thank you, Jill. I'll ask Bill about that."

Enter Bill:

"Bill, were you not affected at all by learning that you had cancer?"

"Well, certainly I would have preferred that the biopsy results would have showed no cancer. But they did, and there was nothing I could do—or needed to do—about it in that moment."

"Since reading Eckhart Tolle's book, *The Power of Now,* I no longer create drama in my life. Also, I have learned to live in the present moment, not the past or future. On page 150, Tolle discusses the end of drama in our lives. And in this moment, I was enjoying my session with Jill and I was ready to get back to it."

"Bill has obviously been greatly influenced by Tolle's book. In fact, he now teaches a class based on the book. I was able to speak to Mr. Tolle via satellite."

"Mr. Tolle, this is Walter Cronkite. Can you explain why Mr. Raines was so calm when he received the biopsy results?"

"Obviously he knows the difference between his life and his life situation."

"My fellow Americans, I don't have the faintest idea what he means by that. Yes, but it was a diagnosis of cancer. Wouldn't that be a little unsettling, Mr. Tolle?"

"Well, it is what it is. One does not need to make a problem out of it, as I point out on page 54 of my book."

"I am reminded of the statement, 'It depends on what you mean by *is*.'"

"To learn more about how the treatment program is going, I speak to the oncologist in charge of the treatment program. Doctor, how would assess Mr. Raines' progress so far?"

Postcards from Oncology

"Well, the radiation bombardment has been directed at the pelvic region for 25 days, and the war is now ready to move into Phase Two. You have to start this war by attacking the outlying areas to make sure that no terrorist cancer cells have escaped the Village of Prostate. Of course, the outlying provinces of Bowel and Bladder come under fire. You can only hope that the casualties will be minimal."

"Recent reconnaissance photos indicate that the cancer terrorists are huddled down in the caves of Prostate Village. After viewing the photos, I can see that we have the enemy nailed down. Now we're going to blast him. From now on, all of our bombing will be limited to the territories of Vas Deferens and Prostate.

"Meanwhile, reports confirm that there is great jubilation and celebration in the territories of Bladder and Bowel. In fact, B and B are throwing a big party next week. Everyone is invited. Bring your own Immodium and Flomax."

"So, with this we leave Arizona and Bill Raines, and the end of the story is yet to be determined."

"And that's the way it is on September 12th, 2003. This is Walter Cronkite with 'Eye on America,' signing off."

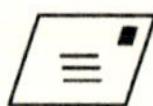

Postcards from Oncology

Along the oncology trail: 9-17-03

Today is my mother's birthday. She would have been 96. This one's for you, Mom. I miss you. You were always terrific for me when I didn't feel well. I know how pleased you are watching the wonderful way Sat Atma is supporting me during this time.

This is Prostate Cancer Awareness Week so I thought that I would drop in to the Oncology Department and pay my respects. The message is, "Get those PSA checkups, guys."

Since it is Wednesday, I get my visit with the doctor.

"Good morning, Doc."

"What do you mean by that?"

"I mean another day in Paradise."

"Okay, Paradise, bend over and let me see your butt. Ah, no redness, no swelling. All right! Damn the torpedoes, full speed ahead."

I call this examination the "Monkey Test." If the butt is not red like a monkey's, that doesn't mean that

I'm not in heat. It means that the radiation has not yet scorched me. If that happens, we will have to take a break from the radiation for a few days.

So I have another blessing to be grateful for in paradise today. It's not red, so it's full speed ahead.

"Well, Sport, two and a half more weeks to go."

"Whatever will I do to start my day, then?"

"We are going to miss having you come around here every day."

"Thank you, it's certainly been fun for me. You folks are great."

Meanwhile, we have a report coming in from the outlying provinces of Bladder and Bowel. Stay tuned.

"This is Walter Cronkite with an update report from the provinces of Bladder and Bowel. Both territories are now fully secure and it's business as usual. The Immodium has been put in storage and the curfew has been lifted. Things are back to normal, and the inhabitants are chanting, "No more soaking, no more soaking."

Postcards from Oncology

Evidently, they have forgotten the clay baths. Some claim that soaking in a tub of water filled with powdered clay draws some of the radiation from your body and reduces side effects. Last week, as I was running the water in the tub, our two cats came in to watch. They seemed fascinated by the sound of running water. I climbed into the tub for my thirty-minute soak. A favorite Charley Thweatt song called "Surrounded In An Ocean of Love" started going through my mind, except the words were different. If you know the tune, please sing along:

Surrounded in a bathtub of clay.
Surrounded in a bathtub of clay.
I am surrounded.
Look around the bathroom, the cats are all in place.
Sat Atma's standing nearby, a big smile on her face.
I am in a bathtub of dirty, dirty clay.
All my radiation is soaking away.
Surrounded in a bathtub of clay.
Surrounded in a bathtub of clay.
I am surrounded.
I am playing in the water till the 30 minutes is done.
I hear Sat Atma saying, "You're having way too much fun."
I have always wanted to play in dirty clay.
I'm in the now moment, and TODAY IS THE DAY.
Surrounded in a bathtub of clay.
Surrounded in a bathtub of clay.
I AM SURROUNDED.

By the way, I would like you to know that Sat Atma never gets to read these postcards before you do, so she has no prior approval rights. She is an incredibly good sport about my foolishness, which is one reason that I married her. However, you should also know that immediately after marrying me she took out an Embarrassment Insurance Policy. I understand that she has recently submitted a claim to the insurance company alleging extreme embarrassment. The Oncology staff is on the list of witnesses to testify against me.

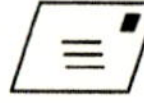

Postcards from Oncology

Another day in paradise, or, "From Oncology to Dermatology." 9-23-03

I drive into the Oncology Parking section, park, and reach under my newspaper on the passenger's seat for my yellow parking permit sign. It is not there. Maybe I threw it into the back seat last time. Nope, not there, either. IT HAS VANISHED. The message is clear: I am not long for this place. As I walk past the receptionist's desk in Maternity the receptionist smiles and says, "I guess I won't be seeing you every morning much longer." Word travels fast.

As I approach the radiation room, Lucy says, "I know, I know, 3/28/27." When they know your birthday as well as you do, you have been around here long enough. As I enter the radiation room, Lois greets me. "Well, short-timer, how are you doing today?"

"Ten, nine, eight . . . but who is counting?"

"You mean you have had enough fun already?"

"I have other ways of having fun besides coming down here and dropping my pants, you know."

"Gosh, I surely hope so, Mr. Raines."

"Is that black crow still hanging around your parking space?"

"No, but there is a praying mantis hanging outside my front door at home."

"I guess there is no limit to the amount of prayer coming in your direction."

"You know, my wife thinks that the praying mantis is cute."

"I see. That helps me understand better why she would marry you, Mr. Raines."

"What am I going to do for abuse after October?"

"We are finished, have a good day, Mr. Raines."

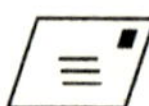

Late September

Off to see my dermatologist. A bonus postcard for all of you readers.

"Come on back, Dr. Raines. (At least here I have some status.) Take your shirt off and have a seat on the table."

"My shirt?" as I pull my pants back up. "Sorry about that, it's a habit, you know."

"The doctor will be right in, Dr. Raines."

The doctor enters:

"Hi Bill."

"Hi Ken."

You know that your skin is in trouble when you see your dermatologist so often that you are on a first name basis with each other. By the way, did you know that the end of my nose was my cheek? Yep, they had to cut away almost all of the end of my nose and they sliced open my cheek and bridged it to my nose.

I hear Wynona singing:

Postcards from Oncology

Love can build a bridge
Between your cheek and nose.
When they find the cancer there
That's the way it goes.
That's the way it goes.

Hey, Greg/Jana/David, I have a great idea for a country western song that one of you could write: "Life Smells So Different Since My Cheek Is My Nose."

Ah, but I digress. Back to the business at hand.

"Bill, this spot on your back is keritosis. I'll freeze it." He sprays it with liquid nitrogen.

"Ouch, that burns. I thought that freezing to death was painless and cold."

"Severe cold burns, Bill. Now, this growth by your knuckle on your pinkie finger looks like a candidate for Mohs surgery. Let's take a biopsy."

Mohs surgery is when they cut tissue away and examine it for cancer cells. If they find some, they go back and cut out some more. They keep doing that until the tissue they examine is cancer-free. As in there ain't no Moh.

Postcards from Oncology

"Call us in a week for the results. If it's malignant we'll schedule an appointment with the surgeon."

"Ah, another visit to Dr. Drummondo?"

"Not on a first name basis with him yet?"

"I'm getting close, maybe I'll try calling him Robert this visit."

"I have a suggestion, Bill. Stop creating these cancers in your skin."

"And how might I do that?"

"Have a serious talk with your skin. Have a good day, Bill."

Later, in my solitude:

"Skin, I have a request. You have created some more cancer. I want you to stop doing that."

"I'm sure. You should have thought of that when you let me bake in the sun over and over for years without a shred of protection."

"I wanted a tan; I looked pasty white."

"What a joke. You, with the red hair and lily-white complexion, wanted a tan?"

"Having a tan makes one more attractive to girls."

"Yeah, but the girls weren't talking about a restaurant for dinner when they looked at you and whispered to one another, Red Lobster."

"That bad, huh?"

"Bad? Remember the 4th of July, 1948? That morning you played 18 holes of golf in shorts with no shirt or hat. Then afterwards, you hung out at the lake for the rest of the day in your swimming trunks. You were so sunburned that night they almost took you to the hospital. So don't be complaining to me now about skin cancer."

"Hey, Skin, that was 55 years ago."

"Well, sir, it takes some time for the basal cancer chickens to come home to roost. Be grateful we haven't created melanoma for you, Bud. You reap what you sow."

Prostate: "Could I get a word in here?"

"You, too?"

"Damn right. If you hadn't acted like a mink in heat those nine years in Saigon, Bangkok, Singapore, Taipei, Hong Kong and Manila, we wouldn't be in this fix."

"Wait a minute. In the first place, why do minks get such a bad rap about their sexuality?"

"Have you ever been around minks?"

"No."

"Well, if you had, you wouldn't be asking."

"More importantly, surely all those years have nothing to do with this cancer?"

"Oh really, do you think the tooth fairy put the cancer in me? Check it out in Louise Hay's book, *Heal Your Body*. Page 58: 'Prostate problems can be caused by sexual pressure.' Nine years of daily pressure, my man. What do you think that did to our level of immunity? For every action there is a reaction. Physics 101, Bill."

"Okay, okay, okay. I'm living consciously NOW!!"

Skin and Prostate: "Indeed you are. Better late than never. We appreciate it, and we all may get to stay around longer because of it."

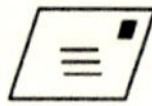

Another postcard from Oncology
9-24-03

And what day is Wednesday? It's "See The Doctor Day" at Oncology. I will spare you the account of our usual foreplay of these visits and get to the nitty gritty.

The doctor enters with his familiar greeting, "Hi, Sport."

"Hi Sport, yourself. So what are the chances that the cancer will be eliminated when I complete treatment next week?"

"Zero."

"Zero?"

"Zero!"

"Then what have I been doing here the past eight weeks, beside keeping your staff amused?"

"If we took a biopsy today we would find cancer, the same as when we started. The radiation changes the DNA of the cancer cells so that when they divide they cannot produce any more cancer cells. Eventually these will die and be no more."

"I had the vision of all of these dead cancer cells lying dead on the battlefield of Prostate Territory."

"It doesn't work that way, Sport."

"So what are the chances that we can expect a cure here?"

"Quite good, I would think, although there is no guarantee. The odds are definitely in your favor. We're done, Sport. There is another doctor here to see you. I'll leave you two alone."

"Mr. Raines, I'm Dr. Holsum. I'm a staff psychiatrist and the folks in Oncology asked me to stop by and have a chat with you."

"About what?"

"Two things that go hand in hand. Mr. Raines, are you familiar with the concept of denial?"

"Indeed I am. I see a lot of that in my work."

"Well, Mr. Raines, from reading these postcard emails in your chart, you seem to think that having cancer and getting radiation is one big joke. You acknowledge no fear and show no worry. They report that you show up here every day like you are going for a stroll in the park. This is not normal for a cancer patient, Mr. Raines."

"I am not interested in being part the norm, doctor, I shoot for higher than that."

"But prostate cancer is life threatening, Mr. Raines, it is not a joking matter."

"It is birth that is life threatening, doctor, not cancer."

"Birth?"

"Yes, when we are incarnated into our bodies we get a coin with two sides. One side is birth and the other side is death. We can't have one without the other. Physically, we are born to die, doctor. However, our spirit is eternal. Actually, it is a wonderful arrangement when you think about it. As the Buddhists say, 'No self, no problem.'"

"Well, what about WHEN you die, Mr. Raines? Cancer can shorten your life, you know."

"Doctor, my time on earth will be just the right length for me. It will be perfect, absolutely perfect! Already, I've had 20 more years than John Ritter."

"Well, what about physical pain and suffering, Mr. Raines? Are you calm, cool and collected about that, too?"

"Well, Doc, at this time I am not suffering or in physical pain. So that is not currently a problem, as I see it."

"WELL, DAMN IT, YOU JUST MIGHT BE IN THE FUTURE."

"There is no need to raise your voice, doctor. Are you under a lot of stress? You seem rather tense."

"You have no idea, Raines. Sick and dying people all day long—I sure as hell can't cure them. I feel so helpless. I work in this environment of sickness every day."

"That must really be tough, Doc. But you know, just the fact that you spend time with them and listen to their concerns and feelings surely counts for a lot."

"You really think so?"

"I'm sure of it. Yet, it must be a great relief when you leave here and go home at night to be with your family."

"If that were only so, Raines. Things are not going well on the home front at all."

"Really, what seems to be the problem?"

"It's my wife, she shows very little interest in me these days. I think maybe there is another man in the picture. In fact, I'm sure of it."

"That must be painful. I hope you have supportive friends."

"No one very close that I can confide in. I just have my work, Raines, and it seems quite bleak to me. Besides, it is not a good idea for a psychiatrist to go around talking about his personal problems."

"The most important thing is to be gentle with yourself. Stay off your case and on your side. I can see that you are a good person. We are all only human and I'm sorry for your pain, Doc."

"Well, thanks for that, Mr. Raines. Now back to you. I am going to schedule you for another hour next week. We need more time to explore this denial issue or yours."

"I look forward to it, Dr. Holsum."

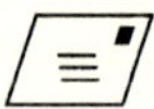

...and the next day at Oncology
9-25-03

Today was extra special because Lucy, Lois and Pat were all in attendance for my radiation. We did a dance called the DNA Shuffle. Swing and sway, while we change your DNA. Swing and sway. Sammy Kaye would have loved it. If you don't know about the big band music of Sammy Kaye you are too young to be my wife. I hope that Sat Atma knows. Oh God, I just asked her and she has never heard of Sammy Kaye. GENERATION GAP ALERT!! We are in big trouble here.

At the end of our session, Lucy said, "Dr. Holsum would like you to stop by his office, Mr. Raines."

Bill, upon entering Dr. Holsum's office:

"Eh, what's up, Doc?"

"Your Bugs Bunny impersonation is not very funny, Mr. Raines. I suppose you'll be showing up in a clown costume tomorrow?"

"You mean like Patch Adams? You know he is a real doctor?"

"Yes, but some of us live in the real world, Mr. Raines. How ridiculous would it be for me to come to work in a clown costume?"

"That would be a tough sell for a psychiatrist, Doc. No doubt people want you to take their problems seriously. It is a disease of the human mind, don't you think? Why are we meeting today? I thought that we were going to meet next week?"

"Well, Mr. Raines, you only have one more week here and I decided that it is definitely going to take more than one session to get you out of your denial. Today I want to talk with you about your repressed anger."

"Anger? Do you see any indication that I am angry, Doc?"

"None whatsoever, and that is exactly why I know that you are repressing all of it. Repressed anger is very damaging to the body, Mr. Raines. Don't tell me that you have never had the thoughts of 'It isn't fair' or 'Why me?' since finding out that you have cancer. Everyone has those thoughts when they find out they have a life threatening disease."

"I'm telling you, Doc. Neither of those thoughts ever crossed my mind. Not one time."

"That's not normal, Raines."

"We covered that yesterday, Doc, about being part of the norm. It's not for me. I aspire to vibrate at a higher frequency than that. Much higher."

"Well then, what DO you think about having cancer?"

"I see that it has been a terrific opportunity for spiritual growth and also a great blessing in many ways."

"A blessing? Having cancer is a blessing? That is exactly the kind of comment that tells me that all is not right with you, sir."

"Well, I now have much more credibility with my clients and students when I teach the concept of celebrating life, no matter what. If they can see me doing that in spite of having cancer, maybe they, too, will believe that they can live peacefully in the Joy Vibration, no matter what is on their plate."

"Joy Vibration?"

"Yes, we all operate on the level of either the Joy Vibration or the Fecal Frequency."

"Fecal Frequency?"

"Yeah, that is when you have your optic nerve attached to your anus and you have a crappy outlook on life. Cancer is just one more thing to have an outlook on, Doc. Joyfully seems to be the better choice, wouldn't you agree?

"Hmmm!"

"You know, one of our affirmations at Unity is "I am here to shine the light of my heart on those longing to be more light-hearted. I've been doing that with my postcard emails."

"And I suppose that you view me as one of those people, Mr. Raines?"

"Now that you ask, Doc, I do observe you to be joyless. But I know that inside there is a part of you that longs to be more light-hearted."

"Raines, how can you expect me to be joyful in the face of all the pain and suffering that I see?"

"Well, it is a challenge, for sure. I don't expect it of you, but it is an option. This world is full of pain and suffering, hate, violence, war, illness and much darkness. We can either curse the darkness or shine some light. I've made my choice."

"Who do you think you are, the man from La Mancha? Do you think that you can change the world, Raines?"

"I do believe that I can make a difference where I am. Right now I'm with you."

"And so you think that you can just walk in here and LIGHT UP MY OFFICE?"

"You're raising your voice again and you seem angry. I just hope that your day is better as a result of our time together."

"WE ARE HERE TO EXAMINE YOUR DAY, NOT MY DAY, MR. RAINES."

"If you were really honest, Dr. Holsum, we both know you called me back today because you felt better after we talked yesterday. Good for you. You have a lot on your plate and I suspect that you have no one that you can talk with about it. I am honored that you confided in me. I want to be a positive experience in your life. The staff here is helping to extend my life. It feels good to be able to give back something if I can."

"Psychiatrists aren't supposed to have problems."

"Sure they are. You are human just like everyone else. Once I was in a therapy group for therapists. It was great. And my clients and students just love it when they hear that I am not handling something well. It makes it easier for us to bond. We are all in this together, Dr. Holsum."

"Well, I will admit, Raines, you did intrigue me yesterday and I did want to get to know you a little better."

"Likewise, Doc. Maybe we could chat several more times before I finish my treatment. No doubt I can pick up a few pointers from you. Just call me Bill."

"I'd like that, Mr. . . . er, Bill. Could you drop by tomorrow after your treatment? And call me Marcus."

"As in Welby? Tomorrow, Marcus, I'm meeting a dear friend for breakfast at 9:00. How about Monday?"

"OK, Bill, see you Monday."

"Have a great weekend, Marcus. I'm sure that I will."

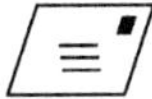

Oncology News Flash: 9-27-03

At 7:00 a.m. Friday morning the phone rang at the home of Bill and Sat Atma Raines.

It was Lois from Oncology, canceling Bill's radiation treatment. It seems that "the machine is down again." I am sure that all of you remember the last time the radiation machine refused to work because he felt rejected by Bill. Time to check back with RM.

"Hey Dude, what's up that you weren't working yesterday?"

"Hi, Bill, did you enjoy your breakfast with Carla?"

"Of course, hey, wait a minute, how did you know that I had breakfast with Carla on Friday morning?"

"One mind, Bill, remember? One mind in God. I heard her ask if you could meet her earlier than 9:00 a.m. Well, I knew that you could not if you had to see me at 8:30."

"RM, don't tell me that you faked not being able to work so that I could make an early breakfast with Carla?"

"Well, Bill, let's just say that it seemed like a good time to give all my clients a nice three-day weekend. You didn't answer my question, Bill."

"You bet, I had a terrific early breakfast with Carla. You are way cool, RM."

"Yeah, and now you know that I don't just kill cells, I alter DNA. I'm glad that you know about that. I have such a bad reputation, Bill. I don't deserve it."

"Yeah, RM, I now see your work in a whole different light and I've been getting the word out."

"I appreciate it, Bill."

"Hey RM, whatever developed between you and that attractive lady machine upstairs? People ask me about that a lot. You do seem more upbeat than before."

"Dude, you were right. That Cat Scan machine is some fox. I just got a poem from her, too. Would you like to hear it?"

"You bet."

Postcards from Oncology

To RM:

You are down there.
And I am up here.
But when you beam me your energy,
I feel you very near.
I take the pictures
And show you where to aim.
You radiate those cells
And the DNA is never the same.

You take care of your business
And I'll take care of mine.
I like your energy, dude,
Will you be my Valentine?
Scanning you,
Cat

"Wow, RM, that's great. I'm so glad that you don't feel so isolated now."

"Thanks, Bill. By the way, the word is out on the machine grapevine that Holsum is vibrating at a different frequency these days. You know, a little spring in his step and a sparkle in his eye. You've been talking to him, right?"

"Well, I have been seeing him so that he can help me get out of my denial."

"Yeah, right."

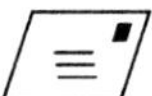

Oncology and the short-timer: 9-29-03

"Good Morning, Mr. Raines, I presume that you did not want to come in for your treatment on Friday. Am I right?"

"Lucy, why would you assume that?"

"Why, because the machine shut down again and the technician could not find a thing wrong with it. The last time that happened you wrote that it was because the machine felt hurt that you didn't want to show up that day. Now I'm beginning to sound as weird as you."

"Lucy, if you start thinking like I do, you and I will be having group therapy with Dr. Holsum."

"Mr. Raines, we have other patients here besides you. We can't have this machine shutting down every time it is inconvenient for you to come for treatment."

"Talk to the machine, not me, Lucy. I was prepared to be here and forgo my early breakfast with Carla."

"Well, I hope that you are prepared to be here the rest of this week?"

"I am, I promise."

"Dr. Holsum wants to see you again. That man has his work cut out for him dealing with you, Mr. Raines."

"I'm sure that he would agree with that. See you tomorrow, Lucy."

"You promise?"

"Yes, and I always keep my promises."

Down the hall:

"Good morning, Marcus, you wanted to see me?"

"Come in, Bill. I am sure that today we can get to the bottom of this denial that you suffer from. I've been thinking about you and I am quite sure what's underneath this. As a child, you were never permitted to express anger. Am I right?"

"Bull's eye, Marcus. My dad never tolerated me expressing anger even when he spanked me."

"I KNEW IT! Now what about crying, was that accepted by your father, Bill?"

"Absolutely not. The message to me was don't be a baby or a sissy. And, if you cry, I'll give you something to cry about."

"EXACTLY! So no doubt you are this bundle of repressed anger and sadness regarding your cancer. I see why you are so stoic about it all."

"I am not stoic, Marcus. I am peaceful. There is a big difference. Besides, I may not even still have cancer, Marcus."

"What? How could you not? Your treatment isn't complete!"

"Well, in addition to my radiation, I have two people who have been doing hands-on healing. Plus, I have been the focus of group chanting several times."

"And what exactly do they chant?"

"Ra Ma Da Sa, Sa Say So Hung."

"So Hung, Bill? Listen. I have heard the scuttlebutt going around that . . ."

"Stop it right there, Marcus. In this context, these words represent the healing energy of the Universe. Others have been chanting that and focusing it toward me."

"So, if you think you're cured, why are you still doing radiation?"

"Well, I made an agreement with Doc to do 39 or 40 treatments, and I like to honor my contracts. Besides, it is a good precaution to complete the treatment."

"Let's get back to the business at hand, Bill. I have a bataka if you would like to pretend that the couch is cancer and beat it and scream."

"Thanks, Marcus, but I feel quite peaceful this morning. I really do."

"I'm not getting through to you. I must not be a very good therapist."

"You did great, Marcus. You were right on the money about my childhood. That was very insightful. It just so happens that I am into living the Power of Now rather than focusing on the past or future. This time here with you has been great. In fact, each day is quite wonderful. I'm here for 30 minutes, and I enjoy my time with the girls in Radiation. The oncologist is great fun, too."

"If only I could enjoy my days like you, Raines."

"Ah, the great news is, you can, Marcus. In fact, I'm starting a new "Power of Now" class this Sunday. Why don't you come and check it out? You'll meet some fantastic people."

"Maybe I will. My wife is moving out and I don't have much else to do."

"Check my website, www.billraines.net. It has all the info, Marcus. See you on Sunday. You'll be in an ocean of love."

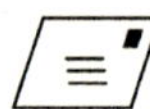

Another day in Paradise, especially at Oncology.
10-3-03

I am walking down the hall at 8:15 a.m. on my way to the waiting room. Lois and Pat come up from behind me, one on each side, locking their arms in mine and turning me toward the radiation room.

"Off we go, Mr. Raines."

"Into the wild blue yonder" (me singing)

"Flying high into the sun" (them singing together)

As the three of us arrive in the room:

"You know, you gals are really terrific."

"Yes, we are!"

(Lois, smiling) "Just kidding."

"Don't discount it, Lois. Claim your magnificence. All of you."

"Ok, if you say so. We claim our magnificence." (Lucy)

"As do I. My wife and I are having breakfast when I finish here today. She is here getting physical therapy on her back."

"How long have you been married, Mr. Raines?"

"Fifty-two years."

"Wow, congratulations. Very few couples stay together that long anymore."

"Sat Atma and I have only been married thirteen years. I have four ex-wives that account for the other thirty-nine years. I've been married five times."

"Mr. Raines, you are joking. Tell me you are joking."

"No, this is my fifth and last marriage."

"I've never met anyone married five times."

"Well, there's Liz Taylor, Zsa Zsa Gabor and me. Actually, the fifth time is the charm."

"Thanks, Mr. Raines, but I think I'll pass on that idea. Here's your chart. Enjoy your visit with the doctor."

A little later:

"Doc, what a soft gig you have. Meeting patients a few minutes every week to hand out a little abuse."

"Right you are, Sport, drop 'em and bend over . . . looks fine."

"You know, Bill, you do that with a certain flair. I think it is in your nature to moon people."

"Yeah, and my opportunities are so limited. When I try it with Sat Atma, all she asks is if I have anything new to show her?"

"Sad to have a flair go to waste, isn't it? Well, you have two more days of radiation, Sport."

"So this is my last visit with you?"

"Not exactly, I want you to return in four weeks and I will digitally examine your prostate."

"Wow, now this is what I call planning fun for the future."

"Well, it will give you something to look forward to for the next month."

"I'll think of nothing else."

"It has truly been great fun having you around here on a regular basis for the past two months. Your energy helps to lighten things up a bit around here."

"Thanks, Doc, you and your gals surely provide an environment that makes it easy for that to happen."

Later when having breakfast with Sat Atma:

"Bill, you really enjoy your time with those people, don't you?"

"You're going to miss them, aren't you?"

"Without a doubt."

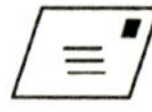

Dear Lucy, Lois and Pat, the radiant gals of Oncology,

I am writing to express my gratitude for the most wonderful way that you have provided my radiation treatments these past 8 weeks. You have gone about your job in a most professional manner. I can only just assume that you all know what you are doing. :-) Trust is a wonderful thing, isn't it?

In addition to that, you three have been simply delightful fun to hang out with for a brief time each morning. All of us cancer folks are blessed to have such pleasant, upbeat, and friendly radiation therapists. Not only that, I believe that the work that you do has added more years to my life. I help people in my work, too, but it is not a life and death situation, more like miserable or joyful.

Attached are the most recent copies of my Oncology Musings. I plan to publish them in a book so that people can see that it is possible not to be so serious about this experience of radiation. I promise to explain that all of the conversations with you three are a fictitious product of my imagination. I have even changed your names to protect the innocent.

When the book is published the three of you will get a copy for sure.

Also attached is a gift certificate for a dinner at Mimi's Cafe. When you are enjoying a wonderful meal there (their corn chowder is superb), remember that you are appreciated for what you do and even more for who you are. This is a very small token of my appreciation for what you have done for me. If I can ever be of service to you, please let me know. With love and blessings to you and your loved ones,

Bill Raines

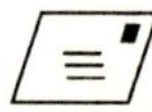

Postcards from Oncology

A Day To Remember... at Oncology. 10-3-03

My final radiation treatment is today. Charley Thweatt stayed at our house last night. He is driving a rental car. It is a gray Alero with California license plates. Why am I mentioning that? As I drive into the hospital parking lot, next to my space is a gray Alero with California license plates. Angels, angels everywhere we turn if we will notice.

As I enter Oncology, I pass the second oncologist's office. He is sitting at his desk. I interrupt to say good-bye and thank him for my opportunities to moon him. The pleasure was his, he tells me. His farewell of wishing me well was very heartfelt. This is a kind, sweet man.

My main man has not come in today. Scuttlebutt is that he isn't good at goodbyes and copped out. Oh well, we have THAT date in four weeks.

"Mr. Raines, come on back." My 39th and last time to hear that. I walk into the radiation room giving the girls my best rendition of Neil Sedaka's "Breaking Up

Is Hard To Do." "Don't take your radiation away from me."

I can tell the girls are very appreciative of my letter of gratitude and gift certificates.

"Mimi's Cafe! I love eating there. Have you tried their pot roast, Mr. Raines?"

"Indeed I have, it's delicious."

"We want an autographed copy of your book, promise?"

"Absolutely, and I will refuse to go on Oprah's show unless she flies all three of you in for it."

"Yeah, you had better treat us right. We know about parts of you that are better left unrevealed to others."

"Not all that impressive, however."

"Pat, did you have to add your two cents worth? All I can say to that is, (breaking into a chant) I AM THAT I AM THAT I AM THAT I AM."

"You are irrepressible, Mr. Raines."

As the treatment comes to an end, I look up at RM above me and say, "Goodbye, and thanks the job you have done for me. Keep up the good work, and say "Hi" to Cat for me."

"Stay cool, dude!"

As they untie my feet and help me up, Lucy tells me that I have to go whether I want to or not.

"I know, and my understanding is that there is no coming back for seconds no matter what."

"Yes, that is true. Radiation is a one-time deal, Mr. Raines. But I am sure that we got the job finished for you."

Lois is standing beside me. Suddenly we are hugging. Then it is hugs all around. As I start to walk away, Lucy's hand is on my shoulder. "You keep that sense of humor and take good care of yourself, Mr. Raines."

As I am leaving the room, I don't have my shirt fully tucked into my pants very well and Lois is tucking it in for me.

"Are you all set with your follow-up appointment, Mr. Raines?"

"You bet, I'll stop by to see you gals."

As I walk out of the hospital my eyes are filled with tears. Just like they are as I write this.

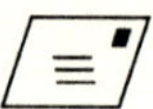

Postcards from Oncology

Further down the cancer trail

10-10-03

On the road again, just can't wait to get on the road again. (Thinking of you, Willie.)

I bet that you were getting worried that you wouldn't be getting any more postcards from me, right? Well, I'm not done yet.

I am experiencing Post Traumatic Oncology Syndrome. I keep waking up every morning at 7:00 a.m. and I have no place to go. Even worse, at 8:30 I beg Sat Atma to put a block between my feet and tie them together. She just laughs and refuses.

Every time I get in my car, there on the front seat is my yellow Oncology Parking permit. I haven't been able to give it up. Yesterday, I did bring myself to throw away the Oncology ID card that I used in the waiting room to check in for treatment.

I go for days now and no one addresses me as Mr. Raines. Sat Atma refuses to do that, too. However, Myrtle Bishop did send me an email and addressed me as Dr. Bill. And absolutely no one is calling me, "Sport" or asking me to drop my pants.

As you can tell, I am really at a loss here. I don't see my urologist again until December. I could try to get my oncologist to examine my prostate earlier than the November date, or I could try to get in to see Dr. Holsum and beat the couch with a bataka. Maybe I could start a twelve-step meeting just for Radiatees Anonymous?

We received the oncology bill yesterday. The bad news is that it was about $40,000. The good news is that I have Medicare. If I had known how expensive it would be, I would have insisted on more than fifteen minutes with the girls each day. My message to the reader is: "Don't get this illness if you don't have good health insurance."

The high point of my life since I last wrote you is that I did get to go in for some skin cancer surgery this week. (Back in the saddle again, out where a friend is a friend. Thanks, Gene Autry.) Sat Atma: "Who is Gene Autry?" (Generation Gap Alert: the alarm indicates that I have married a woman much too young for me.)

The sign on the office door reads: Skin Cancer Surgeon.

Postcards from Oncology

As I walk into the waiting room, the receptionist smiles and says: "Good morning, Mr. Raines." Ahhh, I suddenly feel the adrenaline rush. It seems like old times. However, it is not a good sign that I have been here so many times that she knows me by name.

A little later I hear, "Come on back, Mr. Raines." (It seems to me I've heard that song before; it's from an old, familiar score.) I won't mention the artist because Sat Atma wouldn't know it anyway. *Hint: the bandleader's initials are H.J. and he married a famous movie star whose initials were B.G.*

"Hi Bill, how are you?" (*I told you* that I'd get on a first name basis with him!)

"Hi, Sport."

"Sport?"

"Sorry about that; you aren't my oncologist."

"That's right Bill, so you can stop mooning me and pull up your pants. I'm here to examine your hand."

"That's no fun."

"Well, take off your shirt and I'll have a look at your back."

"It's just not the same."

Dr.: "I want to biopsy this growth behind your ear, and this spot that is not healing on your leg. We already have the biopsy on your finger, so I'll be taking a slice off of there as well."

I watch him slicing on my hand and leg. "Gee, this is just like watching that new program, "Nip/Tuck." It's about plastic surgeons, and they get quite graphic."

"I haven't seen it, Bill, but I have heard about it. We are much more boring since we are not sleeping with one another in this office."

"That's why, you're not a TV series, Doc."

"You've got that right. Go out in the waiting room, Bill, and we'll check this tissue to see if you are clear or if we need to cut some more."

In the waiting room every person has a bandage on their face. The room is full. Skin cancer surgery business is booming.

"Hey, what is everyone in here doing with these bandages on?" (My attempt at humor.)

I get one smile and a lot of strange looks in my direction.

"We could start a support group here and do some bandage bonding." (I don't give up easily.)

More smiles this time and two chuckles.

"I am a therapist, you know."

From the corner: "I thought maybe you needed one."

Laughter all around.

"Actually, I do. I seem to be experiencing some sort of oncology withdrawal."

From the corner: "I rest my case."

"Come on back, Mr. Raines."

"You are clear on the hand, but we need to take some more from your leg and head."

"We've got to stop meeting like this, Doc."

"I was thinking that you could just drop in once every year and just invite me to pick a spot and begin cutting."

As I leave after 3 hours and a third round of cutting, I realize, it just doesn't measure up to Oncology.

The next day Sat Atma is changing my bandages: "Bill, you have a hole on your hand, one on your leg and another on your head. You are taking this becoming a Holy man much too far."

"Holy, everybody is Holy, so Divine, so Divine. Especially me right now."

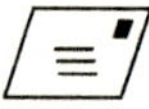

Postcards from Oncology

Follow-up at Oncology

11-3-03

Here I am in the waiting room again at Oncology, one month later. Only the patients have changed. The magazines on the table are the same.

"The doctor will see you now, Mr. Raines."

"Hi, how are you doing, Doc?"

"Some things never change, right? Nice to see you again, Bill. Anything fallen off yet?"

"Out, not off, as in pubic hair."

"You look much better bald all over, Sport. Blame your urologist, not me. It is from the hormone treatment, not the radiation. Turn around and drop your drawers."

"I thought you would never ask."

"Oh, you knew I would. I promised to check your prostate and I always keep my promises."

"Now that you are finished, tell me what you learned from examining me."

"Good news and better news. The good news is that the prostate has shrunk and feels smooth all over. There are no bumps or rough spots. What did you learn from it?"

"I learned that I don't like your finger up my butt. What is the better news?"

"The better news is that we didn't shrink anything else."

"I'm so grateful for small favors."

"How is the waterworks system working?"

"Overtime, I get up every 90 minutes during the night. In fact, I don't even wake up any more. I just sleepwalk my way into the bathroom."

"Sorry, Sport. We have irritated your system and it is hyperactive. I will give you some medication to calm it down."

Next to my chair lies the sports page that I was reading while waiting for the doctor.

"Were you looking at the Hooters ad, Sport?"

"Let's not get into the subject of sex, okay?"

"Sorry, Sport, I understand."

"Are we finished?"

"For today. I want to see you again in two months."

"What for?"

"I like hanging out with you, Sport. There are not a lot of laughs around here, you know."

"I'll make an appointment for January."

On my way out, I stop by the radiation room. Only Lucy is there.

"Mr. Raines, the machine is down again today. I knew that you couldn't be far away. It is great to see you again. Are you doing well?"

"Terrific, tell Lois and Pat that I stopped by."

"You take care, Mr. Raines. When I ate at Mimi's Cafe I had thoughts of you."

"Thanks, Lucy. Bye bye."

This completes the Postcards section of the book. Read ahead for some personal reflections from Bill.

Postscript:

In December, Sat Atma was in the hospital overnight after her back surgery. The next day, when I went to pick her up to bring her home, I had to walk down the hall, past Oncology, to get to the elevator. I decided to stop in to see the radiation therapists.

As I approached the room, there was a lady sitting on the bench in the hall waiting to be called in. I sat down beside her. Lucy came out of the radiation room.

"Mr. Raines! What are you doing sitting here?"

"I was in the neighborhood, so I stopped by to see if I could get a freebie. I haven't had my feet tied up in a long time."

From the lady on the bench: "Take my treatment, I don't mind in the least."

"Mr. Raines, you are as silly as ever."

Pat walks out of the radiation room. "Hey, Mr. Raines, I was absent the day of your last treatment. I didn't get a goodbye hug. Could I have one now?"

"You bet. Lucy, I have one for you, too."

From the lady on the bench: "Dare I ask?"

"You bet, stand right up here." Hugs all around.

"Well, I'm going upstairs to pick Sat Atma up. She had back surgery and she is ready to go home."

"Sexual gymnastics did the damage, right Mr. Raines?"

"Nobody likes a smart aleck, Lucy!"

"You do, Mr. Raines."

"You know me too well, Lucy. I'll see you gals later."

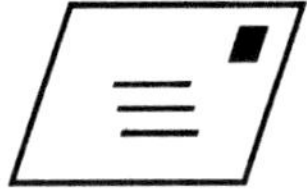

Personal Reflections

We all live from our programming. Our mind is like a computer and we have been indoctrinated from a very early age with core beliefs and ideas that determine how we think and deal with life. In many cases, we may not be conscious of our underlying core beliefs and commitments.

The following five core beliefs are the ones that I use daily to maintain a light-hearted perspective of my life situation. I invite you to consider them as beliefs that can be uplifting and life affirming for you.

The most powerful statement that I have ever heard from a workshop speaker was, "I would know how to behave, even in a concentration camp. "This man was proclaiming that no matter how awful the circumstances, he would know how to respond as an enlightened person. This means that we no longer allow the circumstances of our life to control us. To achieve this we must become grounded in positive core beliefs and faith that provide us with great inner strength.

Belief #1

Resisting what is out of my control is not helpful; it is self-defeating.

Not only that, it creates stress and suffering. Every person who has ever been to an AA meeting knows the Serenity Prayer. "God grant me the serenity to accept the things I cannot change; courage to change the things I can; and wisdom to know the difference."

That is a great, great prayer. However, it would be even greater if we changed it to thanking God for having already given us all the serenity, courage and wisdom that is required of us. Affirming that we have those attributes and applying them beats the heck out of asking for them like a beggar.

The fear-based ego/mind will take one right into the future with some scary mental masturbation. I call it "what-ifing."

Therefore, facing the "what is" of our life and dealing with it with grace, dignity, power and wisdom is the only practical and productive thing to do. Should we choose to sprinkle in lots of humor to boot, our experience of life really gets fantastic, no matter what!

I decided early on not to emotionally resist the fact that I had cancer. At the same time I was committed to being proactive to get cured. Staying out of resistance has surely served me well.

Belief #2

The present moment is all there is.

If you haven't read *The Power of Now,* by Eckhart Tolle, please do. It is transformational. For the past three years I have been teaching a class based on this book. Tolle reminds us that we live our life only in the present moment. The past is dead and gone and the future is never here. It is our mind that leads us to dwell on what has happened in the past or what might happen in the future. Yet all we ever have is this moment, right now!

Most of us "live" up in our heads experiencing guilt, shame and sadness about what did or didn't happen yesterday, last week or last year. If we are not there, we are in our heads showing scary movies in our mind about what MIGHT happen in the future. When we are "pasting" or "futurizing" we are not fully present for what is going on in the moment. Sometimes we are oblivious to the moment and not present at all.

When life gives us a challenge, if we are not conscious the mind will take over our lives. When one is diagnosed with cancer it requires a lot of discipline to live in the present moment each day. What will be the most successful treatment? How much pain is there going to be? What if the treatment isn't successful? What if? What if? What if? That is not my present moment reality. Today, I feel great. I am not in pain at all. I have no idea what the future may bring, but I can celebrate today and do everything that I can to take care of myself. Today, I have the gift of life. I am invited to a feast of joy and peace.

Ram Dass wrote a book called *Be Here Now*. Whenever you start to feel a sense of urgency in your life, check out what is actually going on around you. Where are you? Who is with you? What is happening? Are you being hurt, abused or threatened in the moment? Can you handle what is happening at that moment? Sure you can, in fact you are. Unless we are in physical pain, our suffering is being created by our mind, related to the past, the future or resistance to the present moment. The very best thing that I have done for myself in dealing with the cancer has been to stay centered in the "here and now." We can refuse to create a problem and emotional suffering for ourselves about what has happened in the past or what might happen in the future.

Belief #3
Every day, without exception, I am abundantly blessed.

That is the good news. The bad news is, every day some things will not go the way that I want them to go. For the large majority of us, our minds have been trained to focus on what is not going our way, rather than on the blessings that are showered on us every minute of our day. Even though I have had cancer and I had to go for radiation five days a week for eight weeks, it would take me a mighty long time to count my many blessings each and every day.

Before being diagnosed with cancer I would get out of bed every morning and greet the day affirming, "Another day in paradise." When I started to experience tremendous fatigue and a lot of diarrhea from the radiation, I did not get out of bed so easily. A few days, I hardly got out at all. My mind wanted to trick me into believing that I was no longer abundantly blessed. I wouldn't let it. I still had my terrific wife, more friends than I had time for, wonderful classes to teach, my sight, my hearing, plenty of money … shall I go on? So each day was still another day in Paradise, cancer or not.

For a short time, I did indulge in comparing how much less energy I had during radiation treatment than in the past. I was definitely feeling some self-pity and into some resistance. Then, one morning just before I woke up I heard the voice of Spirit speak to me. The words were, "Bill, whatever energy you do have today, let it be the energy of love." I woke up free of any sadness and I just felt grateful for the energy that I did have. Since that morning, I have been free of any resistance.

A song we sing in church sometimes is, "God is so good. God is so good. God is so good. He's so good to me." And sometimes we sing She instead of He. ☺ Some people report that keeping a Gratitude Journal has changed their life. I'm not surprised.

Actually, many of us tend to be whiners and complainers when things don't go our way. Some of us choose to feel like a victim and to feel sorry for ourselves. "I can't get a break. Why did cancer have to happen to me?" In my classes I pass out an article on what a day is like in the life of Christopher Reeve. I suggest that any student who is feeling sorry for his or her lot in life read it.

I never heard anyone complain in a Ken Keyes workshop about how tough they had it. They wouldn't dare after watching people feed him in the dining room because he was unable to use his arms.

An attitude of gratitude is crucial to being light-hearted.

Belief #4
Everything is perfect for my pleasure or for my growth.

Do you want to get out of Kindergarten or do you want your toys fixed? Most people want their toys fixed. Is that why we came into this lifetime? I think not. We are here to demonstrate that we know the truth of who we are. We are given these challenges to demonstrate that we remember that this planet Earth is not our home. We are just passing through. We are here on our soul's journey in this School of Life on planet Earth. We don't get to have recess all the time. We are like mountain climbers and the higher we climb the steeper it gets. But the view from the top is spectacular. I remember in Martin Luther King's "I Have A Dream" speech, that he talked about his own mortality. He said that he had no fear because he had been to the mountaintop and had seen the view. He was looking death in the eye without fear.

Once we welcome growth opportunities, then we stop complaining about how "hard" or "difficult" things are. If we are never tested, how shall we ever experience our magnificence? So, we can welcome the circumstances that life offers us to demonstrate the best that we have within us. I look at it as moving into an advanced program of spiritual growth. If the lessons are challenging, it must be because we are now in the Graduate Program of the University of Life. ALL RIGHT!!

Belief #5
The ultimate outcome of my life is assured.

On the final page of Tolle's *The Power of Now,* he assures us that nothing we have ever done or that has ever been done to us can in the slightest touch the radiant essence of who we are. That is viewing life from a spiritual perspective. Do you think that you are a human being having a spiritual experience, or are you a *Spiritual Being having a human experience?*

There is no doubt in my mind that I am spirit in form. I know that my body will pass away, but my spirit will not. It is eternal, formless, whole and holy. I believe that the ultimate solution to all of our problems must be a spiritual solution. Anything else is a band-aid.

I am in the Source and the Source is in me. That has always been so, is so now, and will always be so. If I know this in my heart, what is there to fear? When we know this we are liberated from a sense of urgency. There will come a day when I will leave my body behind. It will be like taking off a garment that no longer serves me. But my Self will return to the spiritual world. I am certain that it will be a more glorious experience than this earthly one.

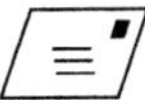

I have offered you five simple core beliefs. They are easily understood. However, living them challenges all that we have in us. I accept the challenge and I welcome it. I invite you to join me in this quest of living as an enlightened soul. Our life is God's gift to us. How we live it is our gift to God. I know that we have free will, but my hunch is that Celebration of Life is the wish for us, operating through the creative force that I call God.

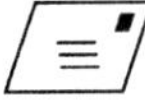

About the Author

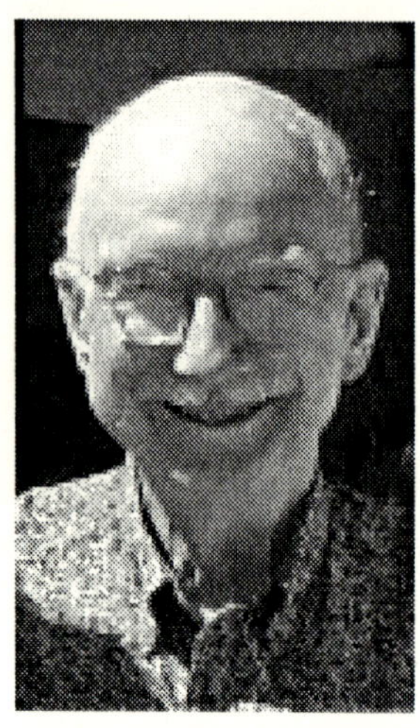

Bill Raines is a Ph.D. psychologist who works from a spiritual perspective. He teaches classes and does counseling at the Unity Church of Mesa (Arizona), and he also facilitates intensive weekend "Advances" (Bill never "retreats") several times each year in the rural and picturesque Arizona communities of Pine and Sedona.

Bill lives with his wife, Sat Atma, and their two cats, Bandit and Casey, in the town of Gilbert, Arizona.

He can be reached through his personal web site, *http://www.billraines.net*, or via electronic mail online at *livlover1@cox.net*.

Postcards from Oncology

For further information or to order additional copies,
please contact the author
or

OPA Publishing
Box 12354
Chandler, Arizona 85248-0023

Or visit the OPA Publishing web sites at
http://www.opapublishing.com/
or
http://www.opapresents.com/

opa

0

WALTRICHARDSONMUSIC.COM

Printed in the United States
19792LVS00001B/97-180